Oil Pulling Therapy: Healing the Human Body through Holistic Means and Oral Cleansing

All rights Reserved. No part of this publication or the information in it may be quoted from or reproduced in any form by means such as printing, scanning, photocopying or otherwise without prior written permission of the copyright holder.

Disclaimer and Terms of Use: Effort has been made to ensure that the information in this book is accurate and complete, however, the author and the publisher do not warrant the accuracy of the information, text and graphics contained within the book due to the rapidly changing nature of science, research, known and unknown facts and internet. The Author and the publisher do not hold any responsibility for errors, omissions or contrary interpretation of the subject matter herein. This book is presented solely for motivational and informational purposes only.

Table of Contents

Introduction

Oil pulling is also commonly known as pulling oil or oil swishing. In many ancient literature it is referred as Kavala gandusha or gandusha. It is type of ancient practice which involves moving oil around in and your mouth in order to remove toxins. In the Internet the technique has become the hit as Internet is filled with loads of reviews and different techniques and usage pattern to provide the complete guide and clarity over the subject matter. In the last couple of decades, the technique has become popular as an easy and effective way to improve oral health without outing up so much of an effort. The actual oil pulling technique is mentioned in Charaka Samhita which is written in 200-400 BCE. This healthy technique is considered to be providing lots of benefits since hundreds of year. It is also being respected technique is Charaka Samhita as one of the best internal medicines that is still actively being practiced by millions of people worldwide. In the ancient Sanskrit literature it is originally written in the form of poetry. The basic purpose behind the poetry is to make it remembered very easily.

Many people confuses with the term as it mislead to the perception of extraction of black gold. But this is not what we are going to discuss. The article is about another oil pulling technique that has been actively followed in India since thousands of years. Many people did not know about this but there are as many as 500 types of bacteria lives in our mouth only, especially in our saliva. That is what causes the plaque formation that resembles sticky film.

So now apart from your daily routine of prayer, taking shower, work out add this technique to complete the morning schedule.

Why It Is So Famous And Popular Method?

It is the one the perfect way to start your day. You will feel cleaner teeth and whiter teeth that before. Also it makes you feel tightened jaws and gums. People often surprised when they got the clear head after sleep and wakes them in better way than coffee, which is worth a trying. It refreshes your mind and gives the pleasant feeling to start your day with lot of energy. It has the ability to detox and to remove the harmful agents from the body. It rejuvenates the mood to bring back the morning energy that is much required.

People often wonder about the term "Oil pulling" in actual it is nothing but the centuries old habit of oil swishing method. The oil is to be swished in the mouth for the longer duration in specified manner. The duration varies from minimum of 15 minutes to 25 minutes also. It again depends on the person to person as what time suits them comfortably.

The Pulling Mechanism

The main theory behind the following of the practice is to that the oil acts as a magnet to attract all the harmful contents. By swishing the oil into each nook and corner of your mouth it collects all the metal present along with harmful bacteria and toxins.

Actually our body produces a lot amount of saliva though out the day. Now what happens is that the saliva along will all other contents also has the bacteria and we swallow that saliva as a natural process. In the oil pulling method the bacteria and toxins are being accumulated in the mouth and attach with the oil. So it keeps the bacteria from being in the saliva and maintains the health of the oral cavity.

The most common practice is being followed in India and that too since thousands of years. There are practically lots of ways that our mouth gets dirty from the simpler habit of chewing the pen when we are into deep thoughts or in the times of anxiety. Not to mention the food we eat has the lot of such bacteria that fills our mouth and gets rested on our teeth and gums. As a result of improper flossing the germs are not removed completely and it moistens the mouth.

The average time we swallow in 24 hours is estimated to be about 1900 to 2100 time, which is looks like enormous number. All the saliva along with the bacterial sets inside the gut they are not being removed. The common cold and flu syndrome has been the product of bad oral health. By oil pulling one can maintain the clean and healthy track records on not being sick in years. Of course you need to have a nutritious and healthy diet along with oil pulling for the best health effect.

The Best Oils Used For The Oil Pull Remedy

Apart from knowing the techniques and the health benefits it is also very crucial to know about what oil to use as it is the main ingredients used. Your freshness level and oral benefits depends on the oil you use. It is also important to know the oil type that suits your body and your need as the same oil can have different types of effects on two persons. Here is the list of oils that used in the technique.

Sunflower Oil

Sunflower oil is very famous for its herbal benefits and it is being recommended in the Ayurveda. It contains the fatty acid that is good for oil pulling. Apart from fatty acid it has 16% of Linoleic, 70% of Oleic, 4.5% of Palmitic and the rest of the portion it contains 3 to 3.5 % of Stearic.

Coconut Oil

Again the commonly used coconut oil has the fatty acid profile, containing 4.5 to 10 % of Caprylic 6 to8 % of Capric. Its most of the part contains of Lauric which is present almost 45 to 52 %. Along with them it has 1 to 2 % of Linoleic, 15% to 21% of Myristic, 5 to 11 % of Oleic, 7 to 10% of Palmitic and 2 to 3 % of Stearic.

Coconut oil is being used as it has many properties like enzyme action, antimicrobial and anti-inflammatory. The fatty acids contents present in it completely remove the unwanted bacteria and keep the stains that are probiotic in nature providing the complete exchange solution.

Olive Oil

We all know about olive oil benefits and how popularly it is being used for various health recipes. Due to its fatty acid profile it is being used very in oil pulling technique.

Sesame Oil

In the ancient Hindu Literature it is being widely recommended as a trusted ingredient for oil pulling as it is based on fatty acid contents. It its major portion it contains 45 to 47
% of the Linleic.

Apart from these oils any vegetable oil also will do but the commonly known oils are coconut and sesame as they tend to have great effects. In the mild flavor coconut oils makes you very pleasant experience. Virgin olive oil has got the reviews of being very strong.

The Race Of Best Oil

There is a study reported to be conducted in the group of people to test the oral effects of coconut oil, sesame oil and water.

In the results the group who has used the sesame oil has found to have five times less bacteria that the other two groups. Then they all are being told to decrease the usage of all the oil types and as predicted the level of bacteria has shown to increase after few days.

- There are many warning signs given in the online materials related to the guide of oil pulling in which amalgams are used. It is also knows as metal fillings. The metal can be proved harmful to the oral health as it can leach into your oil. It is also being absorbed by the soft tissue in the mouth.

- There are also many incidents in which metal fillings are loosened. It falls out in most of the cases. Researcher has not been successful in searching for the evidence of leeching out problem. So it is advised that if you have loose and old fillings then use it with gentle care as it can make further loosen out fillings that are already loosen.

- Also warnings are being given in case of using Mercury-based fillings. It expands over the time in the mouth and also has the capacity to break (Crack) the tooth.

- Although to be on the safer side you can add activated charcoal and also Bentonite clay to the oil pulling every day. It is being advised to add as it has the characteristics of absorbing the metals and also it pulls the heavy mental from the body.

- It must be remembered that if you want to get the maximum effect then it must be initiated with the daily diet of Ayurvedic diet regime. The diet enhances the body mechanism to attract more toxins to oil.

The Process Of Pulling Oil

There are basically six steps in pulling the oil from ones mouth, which are described in detail below:

Oil Wash

This is the first step in the process of oil pulling and one can use an array of oil to remove the toxic oil from one's mouth. A person can choose from sesame oil, sunflower oil, coconut oil and olive oil. We have to intake the oil in out mouth directly, so it is very important that we use the high quality oil, which is rich in essential fatty acids. This is the main reason that, the four kinds of oil mentioned above are used most frequently. One should put in some oil in one's mouth at the start of the day, before the start of the first meal, and swish it in the mouth for some time. One should note that for a start one can take in one spoon of oil and can increase the quantity later on. One should not do a rigorous swish of oil in the mouth; rather move the oil gently in the mouth for some time. This will help in working of all the muscles which remained idle for most part of the day. One can even start with this step for 5 minutes and then increase it till 20 minutes, during the daily course.

Pulling Oil From Mouth

It is important to pull the oil in between the cavities in the mouth and also from above and below the teeth. It is very simple to accomplish this task wherein one will have to put all the oil in from of the teeth and suck it from the space in-between the teeth, that is in between the cavities. This process should be done across all sections in the mouth. If it gets troublesome, then one should find some way of distracting one's mind from this process. This particular process is known as "pulling oil" from mouth.

Discard Away The Oil

Now, it is obvious still worth mentioning, that we need to throw away all the waste oil in some box or some dustbin. It is advised that one should not throw the waste oil in wash-basin because it will get stuck in pipes and will cause problems in later course of time. The oil hardens once thrown away, and it will not move down the lane easily. In no circumstance, one should swallow that oil because that oil contains all the toxic material, which was suck out from the mouth. If that oil goes inside our stomach, then it will cause of troubles to our digestive system.

Brush The Teeth

Even if we have removes out all the toxins from our mouth, it is important to brush the teeth with the normal toothpaste, which we use in daily routine. This will ensure that we have cleaned the teeth even more properly, from all the angles. One need not use some special kind of toothpaste in this case, as the oil pulling process does not leave some after affect in the mouth. However, if one has sensitive teeth, then they can go for the toothpaste those are clinically proven for the sensitive teeth.

Floss

Floss is a very important step in the overall teeth protection and oil pulling. Floss actually is a thin nylon or plastic thread, which is used to remove the small food particles that get stored in the cavities of the teeth. Such small food particles are hard to remove while brushing, and that is the reason we use floss in between all the teeth to ensure that no food material is left over in the teeth. One should take special care while carrying on this process; otherwise it will damage the gums. One should also take care that floss is done in-between all the pairs of teeth, and also at the back side of the teeth. For every new set of teeth, new floss is taken and one should not use the same floss for the whole process.

Final Mouth Washing

At the end of the process, it is important to wash the mouth with clean water, properly, so that it gives a perfect finishing touch to the whole process. One should swipe the layer of water, across all the corners of the mouth, and through all the gaps in-between the teeth. This will ensure that all the waste oil, food, and any other substance is finally thrown out of one's teeth and mouth.

The Benefits Of Amazing Oil Pulling Technique

The best and ideal time for oil pulling technique is before lunch time or before any meal time. It is also commonly carried out on empty stomach for the best results.

Save From Bad Breath

Have you ever experienced bad breadth, when you stand beside someone! This basically happens because of lack of proper care given to teeth. After we intake food, then the oil present in food gets stuck to our teeth. Even small food particles gets stuck in between our teeth gaps, and becomes a reason for bad breadth. When we carry on the process of oil pulling, then all such waste material is removed from our mouth and then our mouth does not smell bad.

White Teeth

There is one term used for the degradation of teeth and that is "plaque". When a thin filament gets deposited on the top of our teeth, which has no color per-say, that particular film is known as plaque. This particular film is not removed very easily form our teeth, even if we do a regular and proper brushing of our teeth. When this layer gets deposited at the bottom line of our gums, then it reinforces the activities of the bad bacteria in our mouth. Now, oil pulling is one technique, with which we can crack that particular layer, and clean the teeth in actual terms. When this particular layer is removed from our teeth, then our teeth becomes white and shiny.

Helps Heal Gingivitis

Gingivitis is a common problem faced by many people, which is cause with the activities of bad bacteria in our mouth. When our teeth have a layer of plaque, then it helps in growth of bad bacteria, which in turn disturbs our whole oral system. Their activities disturb the gums and thus cause inflammation in our gums. This particular inflammation is known as gingivitis. When gingivitis occurs, it leads to forming of gaps in between teeth and the gums, because of which the grip of gums on our teeth decreases. This makes the teeth weak. If we undergo the process of oil pulling, then it will help in removal of bad bacteria from our mouth and, will prevent many of our teeth problems like gingivitis, loose gums, and etc.

Facial Muscle Exercise

To get a proper and toned facial muscle, it is important to give them a regular massage and make use of them. When we undergo the process of oil pulling, then we stretch a lot of our facial muscles in this process, that too for a good amount of time. This helps in exercising those muscles, which otherwise do not work much. This keeps our face toned and bright.

Better Health Management

When we eat food, then along with food, a lot of bacteria go into our digestive system. This is really harmful for our body, as it cause various kind of digestive problems and can also become a cause of heart attack for a few. So, it is very important that we do the process of oil pulling diligently from our mouth, so that all such harmful bacteria is removed from our mouth and do not damage our system.

Oil Pulling And Weight Loss

There is no direct study that links the oil pulling with the weight loss. If you believe in the anecdotal evidences then it certainly mentions about the detox effect.

Side Effects Of The Technique

We all know that it has the detox effect on our body so it may lead to some bad effects with the health. People have experienced the following signs of problems

- Running nose and sore throat are the common problems faced by individuals. Also sometimes they have experienced sinus drainage.

- Many have complained about disturbing the sleep pattern after they have noticed the difficulty to wake up from sleep.

- Mild degree of fever is quite common. And also acne has been the one of the commonest in symptom list.

- As it contains the high portion of MCT, in another term Medium-chain-triglyceride. It could lead to the effects similar to hangover in some people with mild headache and difficulty in finding the rhythm for some time after wake up.

- People have experiences the periods of rashes after wearing a metal or jewelry objects.

- If people are allergic to smell of the particular oil then there are chances of vomiting and dizziness also. If that happens one should consider to change the oil as there are many options available and if that continues to experience then one has to recheck the method to confirm that they are following the correct technique.

- It is very common to feel different in the mouth and sometime s people feel to have change of taste in whatever they eat. The technique does not alter the taste in any form, one should let their body adjust to the technique and should wait for some days time.

Do Remember To Always Spit In The Trashcan As In The Sink It Cause The Clogging Problems. Experts Have Stated That Although It Serves Great Health Effects It Should Not Be Used As An Alternative To Treat Oral Problems Or In The Treatment Of Cavities.

Does The Remedy Actually Work?

As thousands of videos and online information are being made available for the readers, people have seems to be showing more interest in the conclusive science. Although it lacks many medical studies and reports from trusted organization, the technique is gaining more and more popularity. Shailene Woodley has recently quoted as she has benefited a lot from the oil pulling and she also mentioned that her energy level during her works has been increased since she started the technique.

Every month thousands of videos are being uploaded mentioning the health effects and usage techniques of it and it is generating the reliability and trust in the usage method. In a formal interview media informed that she was suffering from the kidney problems and then she started to use this method about six years ago. Before that she did not have any medical background, after the failure if the treatment from her doctors this method came to her rescue. She now almost continued doing this the first thing in the morning.

While on another side a famous consumer advisor and periodontist claimed that there is nothing that he found antimicrobial in nature and he just felt the freshness and lightness in the mouth but nothing more. He further advised that bad breath and other oral problems are not necessarily treated by oil pulling. It is advisable to know the basic problem first.

Listen To The Modern Science

To get to the conclusive result a study is being conducted in which 20 students are being divided into the group of two.

The first group is been given the regular mouth wash Chlorhexidine. It is very famous for its anti-plaque and also anti gingivitis properties. They are being asked to gargle for 10 minutes every day.

While another group is being asked to use sesame oil and the time duration for gargles was remained the same of 10 minutes. With the surprise in both the groups the results are the same. Both the group has showed the great immunity level and fighting ability against the germs.

In the similar studies the oil swishing has shown the effect of saponification in oral cavity, especially in the mucosa. The role of healthy gums in maintaining the overall body health is tremendous, it can cause serious heart problems and heart diseases if not being taken care of. That is the reason why many health experts advice keeping in mind to prevent the oral problems.

If germs are not being removed from time to time then it also infiltrate in the blood and can cause serious irritations in the walls if arteries. Interestingly the same germs are found in lot of quantity in the saliva in the heart patients. That establishes the direct connection of heart problems to germs.

In the study conducted to know the real accumulating effect and cleansing effect of sesame oil is being carried out. In the study the amount of level of free radicals and lipid peroxide is tend to be reduced drastically by the ingestion of ghee. That confirms that the oils like sesame helps in the pulling of toxins as it has the lipophilic effect on the oral cavity.

This lipophilic effect is said to be directly linked with the detox theory to pull the toxins.

www.ingramcontent.com/pod-product-compliance
Lightning Source LLC
Chambersburg PA
CBHW072016280526
45788CB00005B/2067

* 9 781523 989300 *